GETTING OVER THE BUMP IN THE ROAD

Larry,

The journey you've taken has touched many people.

Thank you for enriching all our lives and being my first Belay lap partner!

Nancy

GETTING OVER THE BUMP IN THE ROAD

Helpful Hints for Cancer Patients and Caregivers

NANCY JOHNSTON TOLL

Library of Congress Control Number:		2016921233
ISBN:	Hardcover	978-1-5245-7251-8
	Softcover	978-1-5245-7250-1
	eBook	978-1-5245-7249-5

Print information available on the last page.

Rev. date: 12/27/2016

To order additional copies of this book, contact:
Xlibris
1-888-795-4274
www.Xlibris.com
Orders@Xlibris.com
754163

Contents

Why I Wanted to Write This Book

Anyone who knows me well understands that I'm not really a people person. I am one of those concrete sequential science teachers turned technology directors who finds great satisfaction in problem-solving, and I have always relied on my very practical nature to help explain and move through life. This does not mean that I'm not a caring person. It's just harder for me to open up and talk to people in person. When I found myself faced with breast cancer and at the same time caring for my mother who had dementia, my world suddenly changed. I knew I wanted to help others, but how could I do this being introverted, systematic, and practical? Writing about my journey seemed a perfect fit.

This isn't a how-to book, nor is it based on anything scientific or medically sound. It's simply a collection of my thoughts as I experienced them with the hopes that others will find it informational, hopeful, inspirational, and sometimes humorous. I know that everyone's experiences with cancer are unique, and no one should assume that they will feel the same way or have the same experiences as what I describe in this book.

Research is constantly producing new methods and treatments. I just hope that from reading this book, you will get a better understanding of just what a wild roller coaster the journey of having breast cancer and being a caregiver can be and that this is OK.

I also wanted this book to contain two parts. The majority of the book is a running commentary of my journey with breast cancer, but I also wanted to include a second section of quick-help comments that includes things no one ever told me and some of the best advice I did get from others. Whether you choose to read the entire contents or just skip to the quick-help sections, I hope that both cancer survivors and caregivers will find something that will help make your journey easier and help you get over your own bump in the road.

This book is dedicated to my beautiful family:

My husband of thirty-eight years, Denny,
who has always been there for me regardless
of the challenges we've faced;

my children, Christina and Brian, and their
spouses, Jesse and Jenny, whom I only have to
look at to see the love and support in their eyes;

and my three beautiful sisters, Linda, Susan,
and Debbie, who were the foundation of
my support team. I could not have done
this without each and every one of you.

Also to Faith and Ellie who make me
smile every time I see them.

Chapter 1

The Beginning of My Journey

Everyone at my first Relay for Life told me that I would have a new birthday to remember, and they were so right. I will never forget April 12, 2012. It's funny as "2" has always been my lucky number. My daughter was born at 11:22 a.m., my son on the twenty-second at 2:02 p.m., and I had guessed my granddaughter's birthday just a year before on April 22. All of a sudden, all of those lucky charms seemed to be negated by the phone call I got letting me know that my biopsy was positive and that I had breast cancer. That was the start of what often felt like a bad dream that I should be waking up from at any time.

My journey actually started a little earlier in February of 2012. I had been bothered by some diarrhea and was actually very worried that I may have something wrong with my colon. Like many overweight fifty-plus women, I had avoided my doctor knowing that he would tell me that I needed to lose some weight. I have always been one to say, "Just find out what's wrong," though, instead of wasting time worrying; so I did the logical thing and scheduled a colonoscopy which I hadn't had since my twenties. I was very relieved when this procedure proved that I just had a touch of colitis, and there was something I could take to relieve my symptoms. It was on a follow-up visit with my doctor that I just happened to mention that I thought I felt a lump on my right breast.

I had actually felt the lump back in January but often had areas of hardening on and off as I passed through menstrual cycles. This one was different though. I could actually look down and see a difference in my breasts, and the lump I was feeling wasn't changing much over time. My doctor examined me and, though his initial thought was that it felt fibrous and was probably nothing to worry about, whisked me off to radiology for a mammogram. I greatly appreciated the speed at which things can happen in the whole medical field if there truly is a sense of urgency.

The girl who did my mammogram let me know that something was showing up on the image, and I was taken immediately to the ultrasound department. Here I had a student intern along with a male radiologist going back and forth over my breast seemingly a hundred times. They then saved their pictures for the radiologist to look at who actually read the ultrasound images and came in with his verdict: "You have a mass that is not normal, and you will need to have a biopsy."

This was now a little more serious, but again, I can't say enough good things about everyone in radiology and my doctor. They walked me over to the appointment counter where my doctor came out, gave me a big hug, and told me not to worry yet as they won't know anything for sure until the biopsy results are back. My doctor has been my family doctor for twenty-five years and had enough pull to schedule my biopsy that very afternoon. I can't tell you how important that was for someone like me who wants answers as soon as possible. I really don't like waiting.

I wish I could say that my biopsy experience was just as great, but it really wasn't. My husband went in with me as we really didn't know what the procedure entailed, but this seemed to shake the surgeon up a bit. He rapidly numbed the area and told me that I'd hear a click as the gun-like bore was shot into me to drill out a piece of the affected area. Yes, that's what it looked and felt like. I've taken a lot of soil samples with a soil core for science experiments in the past, and it seemed like something very similar was happening to me, yet my skin and tissues didn't like being punctured or drilled. My biopsy was actually one of the most painful experiences of my journey. It didn't help that the surgeon and nurse left abruptly, leaving me to get up and wipe off the blood on my own. I'm usually pretty good with pain, but I was bothered by this body invasion for quite a few days after.

The biopsy process was also the start of what I consider a great problem with our current health care system. A good friend of mine, who had been through this herself, kept telling me, "You have to be your own advocate." I didn't realize what this meant until I found myself having to call the surgeon to find out my results, calling the lab to find out where my results were, and having to line up all of my own appointments. When I retire, I would love to become a patient advocate who helps others get through this process without having to worry about paperwork and test results. All hospitals and clinics should offer a service like this.

I'll describe the obstacles I faced, but I'm sure that reading about them can't convey the utter dismay I had with the health care system at times. Luckily, I met a few caregivers along the way who got me through the process. First, I was told that my surgeon would call me with my test results in a week. Ten days went by, and I hadn't heard anything, so I called him only to find out that the lab they sent my biopsy to had inconclusive results, so they had passed the tissue on to another lab. He was sure I would have results in another couple of days though. Another week went by and still no word, so I called again and asked to have someone call me to let me know what was going on. Finally, I got the dreaded phone call letting me know that my biopsy results were positive.

I was at our Youth Action's offices, helping the workers get their computers hooked up. From that point on, it seems like my life was in a fog for the next six months. I didn't want to break down, as for me, that meant admitting defeat to this thing that I was determined to overcome. I think I did start crying when I got in my car to drive back to my office and called my husband to tell him the news, but my philosophy really was "This is just a bump in the road and I'll get past this." And I do mean that I wanted to get past this, as quickly as possible.

My husband and son went with me to discuss my options with the surgeon who had done my biopsy. From past experiences with relatives going through cancer, it's always nice to have another set of ears when listening to such important information. I lost my father to lung cancer many years ago, and my husband had just lost his younger brother to cancer a year earlier. Sometimes it is hard to remember to ask questions when you're hearing news that will change your life forever. My family is my rock, and having them with me gave me the strength to push through. Don't ever hesitate to ask others to go with you to appointments, or please offer if you can be a caregiver for someone.

I was told that my cancer was considered stage 2 infiltrating ductal carcinoma, but they wouldn't know for sure until they actually removed the tumor. The recommendation was for a lumpectomy since survival and recurrence rate for this type of cancer was considered the same if you had a lumpectomy or mastectomy. I was all for saving as much of my breast as I could, but I wasn't at all confident in having my surgery done by the surgeon who hadn't kept me informed and had caused so much pain with the biopsy. I'm sure everything would have turned out fine having all of my care in my hometown, but I needed to have confidence in the process, and that was lacking a bit. Again, advocate for yourself; don't settle.

At that point, I felt I was really left on my own. They gave me a few phone numbers of other hospitals to call, but I had to call, make appointments, get my files sent to other facilities, and even had to carry my own test results from place to place. Because the original lab didn't have conclusive results, that made the process even more difficult as I had to work with both labs and convince them that I was giving them both permission to share my test results with the surgeon I chose. And finally, I found a saint!

Chapter 2

Surgery

My son-in-law, Jesse, was an athletic trainer (and now a Physician Assistant) and worked with a doctor at Regions Hospital in St. Paul, Minnesota. He also knew a female doctor there who had just gone through surgery and chemotherapy for breast cancer and asked her to recommend a surgeon and oncologist. Being a doctor herself, she had researched the possibilities in depth, and this made me feel very comfortable taking her advice. I couldn't have been happier with my choice.

I decided to have my surgery done at the University of Minnesota, and this is where I found a person who truly inspired me and gave me the hope and confidence that is needed to get through this. Susan was an oncology nurse at the University Breast Cancer Center and really took me under her wing. She called the labs for me when I wasn't getting anywhere with the release of my test results, got me in to see my wonderful surgeon as soon as possible, and told me to call her anytime with any questions I might have. She was so optimistic, caring, and sincere. I immediately felt more relaxed and knew that I had made the right choice. Every cancer care facility needs someone like Susan.

My surgeon at the university was also great. He was intelligent (oh yes, I had checked him out on the Internet) but seemed to genuinely care about me as a patient. He explained exactly what the biopsy indicated and what procedure he would recommend. He did concur with the surgeon who had done my biopsy that a lumpectomy would be the least invasive procedure and would have the same predicted results as a mastectomy. He was also very perceptive and could tell that I am a person who likes to "get 'er done." When the assistant said that the first available date for surgery wasn't until two weeks, my surgeon immediately looked at his schedule and told his assistants he had canceled a conference and that I could get in on the coming Monday. The relief of not having to wait any longer with this tumor growing inside of me was immense.

I'll digress for a minute to let you know that I think I was most scared of not knowing how fast this thing inside me was growing and where it was going to travel if I didn't get it out of me as soon as possible. I could imagine the mutated cells splitting every second and invading my body to a point where I wouldn't be able to get rid of them. None of my doctors really told me how much time is too long to wait, and so my imagination ran wild with this. Then one day, I mentioned this fear to my same friend who told me about advocating, and she told me that she knew some women who had gone months just finding the right surgeon and that waiting one or two weeks wasn't going to be the difference between life and death. I'm sure that some would disagree with this advice, and I'm sure it's also based on what type of cancer you have, but it sure eased my mind a bit, just to have a time frame to relate to.

Even with this knowledge, it was great to be able to get in for surgery as soon as possible. Thus, on Monday, April 30, 2012, the day after my fifty-third birthday, my husband drove me over to the University of Minnesota Fairview University Hospital for my surgery. I have delivered two children and had some minor surgery before, so the pre-op process didn't surprise me much. I was amazed at how many different anesthesiologists came by though. Everyone associated with the surgery came in and introduced themselves to me and my husband, and explained what they would be doing. It was rather comical at times, like a miniparade, and they checked off their name on the chart as they left. It was getting funny until one gentleman came in and explained that I would have a breathing tube in during surgery.

Regrettably, I watch a lot of TV and immediately had visions of a breathing tube being shoved down a patient's throat while trying to incubate them after an accident; or worse, I could just picture a tube being ripped out of a person's mouth after they were awakened. Yes, that scared me a lot. Luckily, they assured me that I would never know I had a tube down my throat as they wouldn't put it in until I was well under anesthesia, and it would be removed before I totally woke up. It also helped that this message was delivered by one of the last people coming through the tiny waiting room, so I didn't really have much time for my blood pressure to rise.

As promised, I didn't remember anything from the surgery. I think I was out before even entering the operating room as I don't have any recollection of what it looked like. I was immediately scared upon waking up though, as my throat was so dry from the tube having been down it that I felt I couldn't swallow. The recovery nurse immediately saw the look of what must have been pure panic on my face and gave me some ice chips to suck on to soothe the tissues in the back of my throat. Oh, did I mention I'm a real gagger too? Any feeling of something in the back of my throat and I'll have an immediate gag reflex, but I'll go into that later in the book.

My only regret from surgery was that my doctor was already in another procedure when I woke up, so I never got to see him again that day. He did meet with my husband afterward and left him with instructions of what I needed to do over the next couple of days. I love my husband and he takes wonderful care of me, but it's not quite the same getting medical instructions from him versus a doctor; sorry, honey. I might be a little biased, but I think my surgeon did a wonderful job. I had less pain after surgery than I had after my biopsy, and he had taken great strides to remove my tumor and lymph node that they tested through incisions that followed the natural lines of my body.

I must say I was totally shocked when I got home and looked at myself in the mirror for the first time. For this surgery, they don't sew you up and cover everything with bandages anymore (or at least they didn't for me). Instead, I had a blue glue or adhesive painted on me to keep things sterile and held together. Thus, my incisions were right there in front of me to see. I'm sure this can be quite earth-shattering for someone who is squeamish around blood and injuries. I have dissected all sorts of things through my science studies, so I actually thought it was pretty cool, just surprising though.

I should tell you a little about what they did in my surgery (as described by my doctor). They removed the main part of the tumor which was just above my right nipple. He made the incision right along the edge of the areola, or darker part of the breast, and then removed some tissues from around the edges of the tumor. The tissue was put under a microscope right there in the operating room to make sure that all of the edges were "clean," so that they could feel confident that they had removed all of the cancerous cells. They also injected a dye through the same duct that was infected with the cancer cells, and they followed the path of this dye toward the lymph glands, so that they knew which ones would most likely be infected if the cancer cells have spread. They then proceeded to remove one of these lymph nodes through a second incision that was about an inch and a half from my underarm and sent it off for testing.

I was able to go back to work just two days after surgery with very little discomfort. I think I am probably one of the lucky ones as I've known women who have had many problems with fluid drainage and pain after surgery. Just note that it isn't always a bad experience. I returned to see my doctor just once after surgery. Because the university is a teaching hospital, my doctor asked if three students could come in while he examined me. I'm not super modest in medical situations. In fact, when my son was born, we invited one of our best friends, who is gay, into the delivery room as he said the only thing he regretted missing in life was getting to see the birth of a baby. The students who came in to see my surgical scars were rather cute. There were two girls, one of which was right up there, looking around and being very inquisitive. Though there was also a boy who seemed clearly uneasy with the whole thing. Hopefully, he'll get over that if he ever hopes to treat women in his medical endeavors.

I think my doctor likes to show off in front of the students as he went very thoroughly over everything they found, and I left feeling confident that he had gotten all of the cancer cells out in that area. I actually felt sad when leaving the doctor's office. I'm hoping to never have to go back there again, but these people were so supportive and kind. I did send an edible bouquet to the doctor's office after this last visit as a thank-you. Susan called and said that my doctor was gloating and carrying it around the office to brag to the other doctors, showing them what he had gotten. He was so funny and cute that way. It may not be foremost on your mind, but don't forget to thank those who help you along your journey. Many doctors and nurses never get to hear this and they should when they have had such a great impact on your life.

Something else happened that wasn't really supposed to, but it did help ease my mind quite a bit. The nurse at the university sent my tumor to California for Oncotype DX testing. This is a test that looks at the genetics of the tumor cells and is an indicator of the likelihood that the cancer has or will spread to other places. The makers of the test say that the results are only valid for breast cancer where nothing has been found in the lymph nodes. Because my lymph node did have cancer cells in it, my tumor tissue should never have been sent in for Oncotype DX testing. I really think that the university or my insurance company may have a research relationship with Genomic Health, who runs these tests, as they proceeded to test my tissue and my Oncotype score came back as a 12 which is very low. Anything under 15 is considered excellent, and I left the doctor's office at the university, thinking that I may have escaped any further treatment. Oh yes, I was wrong.

Chapter 3

Chemotherapy

I was all psyched up. My Oncotype score was low, I was sure my surgeon had gotten all the cancer cells out, and even the nurse at the university doubted that I'd need chemotherapy. I started seeing a pattern: You think the news is good, but you still have to go through treatment, just to make sure. I was so disappointed to get the news at my initial visit to the oncologist.

I had taken the advice of Jesse's friend in selecting an oncologist to work with, and again, she came through with a great referral. My cancer team that took care of me at Regions Hospital in St. Paul was also caring and super supportive. I did have second thoughts after my initial visit. My husband went with me, and my oncologist happened to be from India originally. I think it was due to cultural differences, but we both felt that the doctor spent the whole time talking to my husband and not me. That was irritating, but it did improve during future visits when my husband wasn't with me. My oncologist was very knowledgeable, and you could tell that the others in the office felt he certainly knew what he was talking about and respected him.

I really appreciated that he had actual research documents to show me that supported his recommendation for treatment, even when I questioned the need for chemo due to my Oncotype score. I wasn't willing to put my body through something like this unless I felt it was going to be worthwhile. Don't ever be afraid to ask your doctor for evidence to support what they are telling you. If they can't produce this, see someone else. The prescription he decided was right for me was four sessions of chemotherapy that were three weeks apart.

At Regions, they have you attend chemo class before your first session. I was so impressed with how thorough the nurse was in describing everything that would happen during chemo and what side effects to expect. There were two others in my chemo class. I really felt sad for these other people as they were in class by themselves. My husband attended the class with me, and I am so thankful that I had someone there with me to hear some of the things that I really didn't want to hear. Caregivers, if you have a chance to go to medical visits with your friend or family member, please go with them. It really helped to have someone with me for support. We got a tour of the infusion room where they give the treatments, and I really felt better prepared for my first session after this three hour class.

The thought of chemotherapy probably scared me the most, and I decided to take my sister Susan's offer to travel from Iowa to help me through my first session. I knew my husband and children were also there for me, but I also knew Sue would have my same sense of "let's just get this done" and not be too emotional, at least in my presence. You should find that someone who will give you the most peace of mind at this time and not worry about hurting others' feelings. This time is about you!

I took my prechemo pills the day before my first treatment. The steroid and antinausea pills did a good job in preparing me for the next day. I didn't have any side effects from these pills (at this time). I prepared my chemo bag: puke bucket (movie popcorn container), water, pudding, crackers, magazines, laptop, books, and anything I could think of that could keep my mind off of what was really happening to me.

My biggest fears going into chemo were that I thought I'd be very sick to my stomach and that I would lose my hair. I am very happy to share that neither of these became an issue for me. The drugs they give you before, during, and after chemotherapy help with nausea so much. Be sure to take them when they tell you to, as they told me to stay ahead of any feeling of nausea. I was sure to do this and also tried to snack every two hours so that I never got to the point of being nauseous enough to make me sick. My sister was great in making me eat something, even when I didn't want to, and I think that was a key to feeling good. There were a couple of times I woke up in the middle of the night and had to eat some crackers or pudding or take one of my "anytime" pills, but that was the extent of my nausea.

The infusion room where I got my chemotherapy treatments was set up like a big party room with a circle of chairs for patients along with chairs next to each one for caregivers. They did have some private rooms that patients could use if they weren't comfortable being out with others, but I never saw many people use this option. We mostly just sat around—each one plugged into their IV drip—talked, slept, read, or watched TV. I must say it did take longer than I expected, but they explained that they go slow at first to make sure that you don't have any side effects from any of the drugs they are giving you.

The nurse would come over and warm my arm up with a heated towel to allow the IV to be inserted more easily. Then they started a drip with Benadryl first, again to negate any allergic reactions to the drugs, but I thought this was the best because it definitely put me in la-la land and took my anxiety away. They don't always offer the Benadryl so don't be afraid to ask if this is an option. Next, I had a bag with a steroid which is supposed to help with nausea and side effects, and then finally, they got to the first bag of my chemo cocktail which, for me, was Taxotere with my second course being Cytoxan. I was expecting to actually be able to feel the drugs enter my body and start working, but it basically was like any other IV I'd ever had. Sue and I talked, and I think I dozed off for a while since I was so relaxed from the Benadryl. My first infusion took about four hours with that working down to three for the last one. Actually, it was pretty uneventful so I just kept waiting for something bad to hit me, and it wasn't long before I experienced my first side effect.

I knew the steroids could make you swell up a bit, but my body must have overreacted to them as my mouth and tongue started swelling up when nighttime fell. I must say that was pretty scary for me as I was having a hard time swallowing (that old gag reflex), and I went into a bit of a panic mode. My husband immediately took me to our local emergency room where I thought they would help me out; however, there must have been another emergency that prevented any doctor from checking on me. The nurse stuck me in a room, and we were left there for over an hour. Luckily, the swelling subsided on its own, and I ended up walking out, never having seen a doctor. I know my husband would have gone on a manhunt for a doctor if it had gotten worse, but it left me dismayed that no one ever came to explain what was happening to me. The next day, I called my cancer care center at Regions where they explained that this can be a normal side effect, and I shouldn't worry too much about it. Luckily, that is the only time I reacted this way.

One more thing that you shouldn't be shocked about if you are a woman is the possibility of chemotherapy setting off a menstrual cycle—ugh. Actually, the same thing happened to me after surgery; I started bleeding pretty heavily after both surgery and chemo, to the point where I bled through pads, clothes, and sheets. This was one of those times I had called Susan from the university who had explained to me that women's bodies often respond to trauma by menstruating. Aren't we lucky? Thus, when this happened after chemo, I wasn't surprised, but it was very helpful to have my sister there to do laundry and keep bedding clean for me.

Diarrhea also set in for a few days after chemo. This is also a pretty common side effect, and there really isn't much you can do about it except to drink a lot of water and make sure you snack regularly to ward off hunger and nausea. You will also notice that your excrements, both solids and liquids, will smell absolutely horrible after chemo. Try keeping beside the toilet an air freshener you can wave around to avoid the smells that can almost make you sick to your stomach.

One side effect you can combat though is dry mouth. If you have a chemotherapy treatment that causes your mouth to become dry (not all drugs do this but mine did), try using Biotene. My dental assistant had told me about this, and it provided great relief.

Though some of these things may sound terrible, they were all short-lived, and I actually missed little work during my weeks of chemo. This would be a good time to also mention that if you are working and undergoing treatment at the same time, Family and Medical Leave Act or FMLA will help protect your job if you do have to miss more than your boss may allow you to. I was working in an environment where I was afraid that I may lose my job, and I found out about the Cancer Legal Line. This is a non-profit organization that offers free legal advice to cancer patients. My husband and I attended one of the free seminars they were having in the Twin Cities and were very happy to find out that my job would be protected as long as I was under FMLA coverage. They have a lot of information available to anyone with cancer, and they also have attorneys that will talk with you one-on-one and offer advice free of charge.

My medical team at Regions also consisted of physical therapists who helped me know how to stretch the areas around my breast to prevent too much scar tissue from building up after surgery. They set me up with some exercises to do that really helped my arm and chest area feel better, and they also explained the need to watch for lymphedema. Lymphedema is the swelling of the arm that can occur if lymph nodes are removed on one side of your body. Because I only had one lymph node removed, they weren't too worried about me, but it was valuable information to have so I would know what to do if I did experience anything like this. They still recommended that I get my right arm fitted for a compression sleeve that I could wear whenever I was on an airplane flight. Evidently, the change in air pressure during flying can trigger this swelling, and thus, I went to the specialist they referred me to and purchased my compression sleeve that I continue to wear when traveling by plane.

Regions also has many volunteers and some help out in the infusion room. One very kind gentleman brought in a cute dog for patients to snuggle while getting their IV and a girl came around and gave everyone in the room massages. They really helped generate a spa-like atmosphere for those who really need a little less stress in their lives.

So what else can happen? Oh yes, the hair situation.

Chapter 4

Beautifully Bald

It may seem silly to devote a whole chapter to just one side effect of chemotherapy, but this chapter is about so much more than hair. I know how I felt going into chemo, and I assume this may be hard for other women and some men. I really am not a high-maintenance girl. I've never worn a lot of makeup or worried that much about how I look. The thought of being bald though was constant in my mind until it happened. The nurse told me that it would be between twelve and fifteen days after my first chemo session that I would probably start losing my hair, and she was right on the money. I'll never forget the morning I got out of the shower to go to work and ended up with a handful of hair in my hand. Yes, it does come out by the handfuls.

I don't really remember much about that day other than frantically calling my daughter-in-law, Jenny, who had been a hairstylist in the past, to please come over after work and cut my hair off. I just didn't think I could go through another morning of having it fall out around me. Jenny was so great. She showed up after work with her electric shears and buzzed me down to about a quarter inch all over. I think she expected me to fall apart, but you know what? I made it through, and it wasn't nearly as bad as what I imagined. Before I go on, I also want to mention that my hairstylist downtown had also offered to let me come in after hours, and she would shave my head down for me without anyone around or, if I wanted, my family could come with. This was a very sweet offer, and I'm sure you could ask the same of your own stylist.

This is the big message here: It doesn't matter what you look like. Your friends will still be your friends, and you will be the same person you have always been—with or without hair. Does it have an impact on your life? Oh yes, but not in the ways you might think.

There are two hair situations I had that still make me sad sometimes. These include the reactions of my granddaughter and my mother. My granddaughter was only one when I went bald, but I really thought she'd have fun playing with grandma's wig. Boy, was I wrong on this one. A friend of mine told me about a place close to home where I could get a wig, so I had gotten one that I thought was pretty cute and not so different from my own hair. When I showed my granddaughter how I could take my hair off and then put it back on, it really did scare her. She ran from my bedroom to her mom, and she looked at me so strangely after that. I'm not sure if she ever really understood that it was still me under the wig.

Three years before I had cancer, we had moved my mother to a senior apartment complex in our town so that I could help keep a better eye on her as she was showing early signs of dementia. By the time I was diagnosed, she had gotten to the point where she needed more care, and we were able to get her into an assisted-living area with a memory unit in the same complex. It was an excellent place for her to be as she was very outgoing and loved to be around other people, but it was hard keeping up with visits, shopping for personal items she needed, and making sure her bills were paid. What made me cry the most though was the fact that she really didn't understand what I was going through and why I was bald.

My father had died of lung cancer quite a few years earlier, and I assumed Mom would remember what he went through and would be able to relate me to the same situation. She had forgotten though and looked so perplexed and sad when she gazed at me since she didn't understand what was happening. It was so hard to lose the mother I had always known, even when she was right there in front of me. I think it is much harder for caregivers helping family or friends with mental illnesses than physical problems. It took me a long time to fully understand that my mom couldn't help me since she didn't know how anymore and nothing I or anyone else could say to her would change this. Thinking of the sadness in my mother's eyes still makes me cry, but my love for her can't be broken.

For those caregivers helping others with dementia or Alzheimer's, please don't try to do everything by yourselves. There are others going through the same thing who can give you advice, and do allow people to help you. My mother passed away from a stroke, right as I was finishing up radiation treatments. I was so tired at this point that I had to let others in, and I was so glad that I did. My mother had belonged to an international women's group; and her friends brought us meals, came and sat, and sang to her when she was in the hospice room. I'll never forget how much I appreciated their support, even though I didn't know all of them personally.

Where else can you get help? The American Cancer Society is a great place to start. They have so many things to help cancer patients. One of my favorite things is a Personal Health Manager Kit that is nothing more than a plastic case that had folder inserts to help keep track of all my medical appointments, bills, prescriptions, doctors' orders, and more. It was so convenient, and I still have all of my cancer-related paperwork in mine. You can get one for free just by calling 1-800-227-2345 and asking for one. The American Cancer Society TLC Direct website offers soft hats, scarves, bras, and more for good prices; and they are made especially for cancer patients. I purchased a lot of scarves and hats to wear after going bald, but many would catch short hairs I still had. The scarves and hats from TLC were made so your head wouldn't get too cold or too hot, and they never would catch on my hair. They also have bras for different types of situations, so it was easy to find something that I could even out with since my right breast was now about half the size of my left. I found myself either just going bald or wearing a scarf much more than wearing the wig since it was so scratchy and hot.

Those short hairs that grow back can be pesky, and I found them catching on chairs and pillowcases which was very annoying. One day, I decided I'd had enough and gave my husband the OK to take his safety razor to my head. Oh my, I don't know who was shaking more. He was happy to help but didn't want to nick me. I was picturing a long gash across the top of my head. He foamed me up with shaving cream, and the next thing I knew, I was as shiny on top as any bald person could be. This was so much better, and he continued to keep my head groomed until chemo was done, and I had real hair growing back.

The good: My hair grew back super curly after chemo. I never had curly hair, so I enjoyed the new waves even though they were pretty short-lived. The bad: Initial shaving with a safety razor can make your head sore with razor burns and bumps. My sister Linda had the answer for me this time. She works with hospice volunteers in Florida and thus has a lot of experience finding things to help patients deal with various treatments. She sent me some Burt's Bees baby lotion and baby shampoo that were the best.

The lotion cleared up the sores, and I was once again smooth and shiny.

Don't forget to pamper yourself during chemotherapy. The American Cancer Society also sponsors makeup clinics for female cancer patients where they give you makeup kits and show you how to draw your eyebrows back on. I did lose pretty much all of the hair on my body which was nice for not having to shave my legs, and I can now fill in my brows with the best of them. Caregivers should consider providing care kits that include makeup, scarves, hats, hard candy for fighting dry mouth, and fragrance-free lotions as all of these things are great for cancer patients.

My chemotherapy continued for fifteen weeks, and I must tell you that the treatments tend to knock you down more near the end as your body has a harder time fighting off the chemicals. It would usually hit me two to three days after my infusion, and I had some days where the Taxotere would make my legs hurt so bad that I didn't think I could walk. You can get through this though, and you will be stronger for having done so, both spiritually and physically.

Chapter 5

The Three *R*s: Radiation, Reconstruction, and
Recovery with a Small Dose of Depression

Remember when I said, "You think the news is good, but then you still have to go through treatment?" I had made it through chemotherapy and was thinking, *I've done it!* Then my oncologist tells me that I still need to meet with the radiologist to see if I need to follow up with radiation. Again, my euphoria was quickly snuffed out. This time, I went to the radiologist who was associated with Regions but worked closer to my hometown. I really didn't think it would matter who I saw since radiation is radiation. This time, I wish I had done my homework a little better. Though the location was close that I could go to daily treatments over my lunch hour, my radiologist was less than supportive.

When he recommended eight weeks of daily radiation except on weekends, right away I asked for documentation that would show that radiation would make a difference in my fighting the cancer that I may still have or deter recurrence. The doctor got very defensive, and it seems that not many had ever asked him to produce this type of information before. After that, I felt he always treated me with some amount of defiance and would constantly suggest that I had it so much better than some that I shouldn't be asking questions or complaining. Yes, I know my cancer could have been much worse, and there are many that suffer much more than I did, but doctors should not treat patients like this.

I did put up with him only because I still was worried about holding my job in what I felt was a rather hostile work environment, and this was the closest place I could go for radiation so I could work it into my lunch hour. Looking back on this, I should have probably found a different place and taken my chances by missing more work. It also helped that I only had to see him once a week, otherwise, my daily treatments were given by two very delightful girls.

Before I get ahead of myself, my initial visit with the doctor was rather awkward, as I said, but then they made a mold of my head and arms that would be used to keep me in place during treatments. That really was nothing as they said it was a pillow of soft beads that would form around your head and arms, and they were correct. What they didn't tell me was that those soft beads were then turned into hard plastic in that same shape. The lesson learned—be sure you are comfortable when they make your mold. Mine didn't feel too great when it was hardened, and a couple of times, they put a towel around my neck to keep it from hurting during treatments.

Everyone told me that radiation would be a breeze after chemotherapy. I'm not sure I would agree. Having to drive to treatment every day, getting into a hospital gown, lying on a flat table with my head in a hard mold, and finding out how incredibly tired I got from radiation makes me think I would rather go through chemo again versus radiation. Note: Once you have radiation on one side, you can't have it again in that same area, so I guess I'm clear on this one anyway.

Radiation isn't very exciting. I did take my sisters with me one day, and I think they had more fun than I ever did since they got to watch in the booth and see the pictures forming as they positioned me. I almost forgot about the free tattoos that you get with radiation. I still have the three little dots they used to line me up on the table—a simple reminder that I made it through this.

In the end, my radiologist wanted me to do four booster sessions of radiation with higher power and wider spread. I wasn't having any major issues with the radiation, but I know how harmful it can be for healthy tissue. Again I asked him to provide research that would support this, and I also did some of my own on the Internet. I couldn't find any documentation supporting that this extra boost would lengthen my survival or help keep me cancer-free. Even the article that my radiologist supplied didn't suggest that it would increase survival rate. This is really the first time I went against doctor's orders and refused the extra treatments. My doctor wasn't pleased with me, but I don't think that he really liked me from the start so I wasn't too worried. You have to stick up for yourself sometimes, and I just felt like I had done enough.

I never knew I could be as tired as I was during and after radiation. I would go to work and daily treatments, only to come home and collapse in a chair and fall asleep. This went on for at least six months after radiation, and I really didn't feel like doing any type of exercising in addition to work for about a year. My husband was so good at cooking meals and keeping the house cleaned up. He is a much better cook than I am, but he never complained about how tired I always was and how much he took over.

I think this lack of energy and my work situation led me into a slight depression where I would cry almost every day on my way to work. I knew I needed help, and again, my cancer team at Regions was there for me. I was assigned a whole team at the Cancer Care Center, like every cancer patient at Regions, and this included my oncologist, his cooperating physician assistant, a social worker, the infusion nurses, and a psychotherapist. After one visit with the physician's assistant where I broke down crying, she recommended I talk to the psychotherapist, later to be known as "my psych guy." Scott was amazing. Just talking to someone who isn't personally involved with you can have such an amazing impact on your outlook. Scott only worked with cancer patients, and thus, specialized in the fears and thoughts that go through your head. He was also a cancer survivor himself and could really relate to what you go through with treatments and surgery.

The first time he asked if I wanted to try hypnosis to help alleviate some of my anxiety and stress, I was seriously doubtful. I imagined the hypnotist on stage, putting his patients to sleep, and having them make animal sounds and do crazy things. I was totally flabbergasted by this experience. Not only could he hypnotize me, but he recorded our sessions so I could hypnotize myself by listening to the CDs at home. The calmness I felt was so nice, and the thought that I don't have to like all people I work with and can still be a good person was such a relief. We worked on things like trying to stay calm during the terrible hot flashes I started having with taking the follow-up chemo drug tamoxifen, and how not to feel guilty about spending more time with my mother. He made a true believer out of me. Scott has retired now, but I think I'm good and am a much better person having known him.

Scott also wanted to try a different hypnosis therapy session when I decided to have my left breast reduced to better match the one I had a lumpectomy on. I was very tired of having to stuff a bra on one side to make me look even, and it was quite embarrassing when going to the gym to work out or swim. It had made working out more of a burden, even when my good friend, Becky, sewed pads into all my sports bras for me. I did find some great pads and bras through the Tender Loving Care or TLC non-profit website, sponsored by the American Cancer Society, which specializes in products for cancer survivors. I don't think Scott realized that I had great confidence in the surgeons and doctors and really wasn't too worried about this surgery; after all, wouldn't it be similar to what had happened on my right side? My plastic surgeon assured me that I would have "the perky little breasts I always wanted."

Another shock. My surgery went well, but I woke up to many more cuts and blue glue holding things together than I expected. Evidently, they don't just remove the same tissue that was removed on the cancer side to even things up. My surgeon had raised both nipples to match and reduced the left side breast, but I think that my oncologist had done a better job of leaving my cancer side looking good. Now I had a small dimple on my cancer side and three large scars on my left side. I also experienced the funniest thing after surgery. I woke up one morning and heard this sloshing sound. It sounded like someone shaking a half-empty milk jug whenever I would move. This was so embarrassing yet very funny at the same time. I really didn't want to go to work sounding like this, but I did and also proceeded to call the doctor to ask what was going on. I wasn't able to see my plastic surgeon again since his schedule was so busy, but I did see his assistant and learned that I had fluid building up which can easily happen after surgery. She proceeded to stick a long needle into my breast along one of the scars and extract what seemed like a great deal of fluid. It did provide relief, but my breast filled up one more time, and I had to have the extraction done again before my body decided it didn't need all of this liquid to heal itself.

Though my breasts are pretty much the same size as each other today, I still have a large scar under my good breast and a little dimple on my right side. I am not a very vain person nor have plans to model for a risqué magazine so I am OK with this, but note that it would be wise to seek out a plastic surgeon for reconstruction who is recognized in this area. While being fitted for my compression sleeve to avoid lymphedema, I did have a recommendation from a girl who worked with breast cancer survivors, but this time I hadn't taken the advice and wish I would have now.

Recovering from cancer treatment is long and hard. I had never been this tired in all my life and still feel that I don't have the stamina I had before getting cancer. I have learned to slow down a bit, and I know that daily exercise does help. For loved ones of cancer survivors, please be patient and supportive as it's very hard to understand just how tired someone can be.

Follow-up has consisted of six month checkups with my oncologist, yearly mammograms, and regular visits to my general practitioner. For my long-term chemotherapy, I had been put on tamoxifen which is a drug that encourages the cancer cells to feed off of it instead of estrogen, and then it proceeds to kill the cancer cells. I had to take this particular drug since I wasn't in menopause yet, and the alternative drug requires that you have already reached menopause. They did test me to find out if I truly was in menopause or only there due to chemotherapy. The tests had conflicting results so my oncologist has continued to keep me on tamoxifen. I won't complain and would actually prefer to stay on this as the only real side effects I have from it are hot flashes and weight gain.

I've heard that the other options include these and also muscle aches which I really don't care to have.

My oncologist did give me a study of an alternative course, but it would require a monthly injection to keep me in menopause along with the drug that can cause muscle aches. The study showed a 4 percent decrease in recurrence of breast cancer compared to the use of tamoxifen, but for me, the study was just too small, and many had dropped out of the study due to the muscle aches they had with the other drug. Since then, my oncologist has recommended staying on tamoxifen for ten years versus the initial five years we had discussed, and I have found studies that do support this. I also found some facial antiperspirants online that help keep my face from sweating so bad during the hot flashes, so this I can live with and I plan to go on living for a very long time.

Chapter 6

Caregiving

I am not an expert on caregiving. I only know what I have learned, and I truly hope that I can help someone who is either suffering from a medical condition or has a loved one who needs help. Having cancer opened up my eyes and made me realize how much we need others in our lives to help support us when the road gets bumpy. Please ask for help before you are underwater and also recognize that there are others out there who need your love and support.

Though I had been a teacher for twenty years and had always cared about my students, my first experience with caregiving for a physical ailment is when my father had lung cancer. He never asked for help and even kept his prognosis a secret from his daughters for some time, but my mother finally called and asked us for help one weekend. Dad's cancer had spread to his brain and liver, and we knew then that he wasn't going to make it. Dad did not like hospitals and wanted to stay at home on the farm, so Mom was his primary caregiver. She did have great help and support from Hospice, but Dad had gotten to the point that he really needed 24/7 care.

My husband and I drove down for the weekend as Mom was worried Dad would try to get up and fall, and she really couldn't lift him herself. Luckily, Denny was with me and was able to help my father when indeed he did try to get up in the middle of the night and fell down. At this point, he wasn't my dad anymore. It was so hard to see him look so bewildered, and the morphine that kept his pain in check disabled him from communicating except for the sad look in his eyes.

I never thought I would ever have to change my dad's diapers, swab his mouth with wet sponges to keep it moist, or hold a urinal in place as he tried so desperately to go to the bathroom. He was a very intelligent man and knew that this meant his kidneys were shutting down if he couldn't urinate. He knew he was dying but just didn't want to give up. You take on roles that you never imagined when a loved one is dying, but it is important to be there if you can. We had to return home that Sunday, and about two hours into the drive, we got the call from my sister Susan that Dad had passed away. I got back in the car when we got home and drove back to Iowa. Not only did Mom need support, but I did too.

I'll never forget two friends who made the long trip to my father's funeral that week. It meant so much to me that Barb and Bill showed up. Just having friends and family around can ease the pain of loss. My sister Linda works for a hospice in Florida and organizes volunteers who help terminally ill patients and families. She knows much more than I do about how much one person can do to help others; and my sister Debbie, who worked in a hospital and later for the state criminal investigation lab, also knows how hard loss is for the people left behind.

My second experience with real caregiving came when we realized my mother was suffering from dementia and needed help with day-to-day activities. My mother knew, at first, that her memory was diminished; but she was very proud and did not want others to see this. She visited us for Thanksgiving, and we happened to go to a pet shop for some dog food, and she fell in love with one of the little puppies. We decided that this would be a great companion for her and that we would get the puppy housebroken then bring it down to Mom's house at Christmastime. This was the great awakening for me. We always had dogs while growing up. My dad was an avid bird hunter and raised German shorthaired pointers, and we had a poodle in our house ever since I was little. When we brought Mom her new puppy, Lucy, at Christmastime, she had no idea on how to take care of it. She had set training pads for the puppy to use outside and had no concept of the need to let her out to go to the bathroom.

During this same visit, my husband's brother was struggling with a brain tumor and was in the hospital, so Denny and my son had gone to see him. This left me, Mom, my daughter Chris, her husband Jesse, and my son's wife Jenny at Mom's house. We decided to pass the time playing some games and were all seated at the dining room table when right over our heads, a bat flew up from the basement. I think Chris and I ducked, Mom just sat there not understanding what was going on, Jesse went to open the door, and my daughter-in-law, Jenny, ran up to the open loft where the bat was flying around over our heads, reached out, and hit it down with her bare hand. She proceeded to wrap it in a towel and let it go outside. This made Jenny our go-to person for any future bat takedowns, but it was also another sign to us that Mom wasn't understanding things clearly as I'm sure the bat may have been living there for a few days.

My mother had always been a wonderful cook, but that holiday, she ended up serving a nice roast beef that the butcher had helped her with, a relish tray, and one baked sweet potato to share between the seven of us. This wasn't my mother's standard holiday meal. Poking around her kitchen, I found melted ice cream and pizzas in the refrigerator, moldy food, and many cans with expiration dates well past. We all knew it was time for Mom to have some help—she had forgotten how to cook.

We headed back home to start making plans with Lucy, who is still happily with us and was a true godsent companion when my husband's brother passed away. I am thankful that we lived in Wisconsin as this is where my mother was born and grew up. Thus, it wasn't hard to talk her into moving from the town she had lived in for many years as she saw this as "moving home." We found a wonderful senior apartment complex which is attached to both nursing care and memory care units which she could easily transition to as needed in the future. By that summer, my sister Susan and I cleaned out Mom's house and moved her to where we lived so that I could help keep an eye on her.

Dementia is a truly terrible state. At first, Mom greatly enjoyed meeting for coffee every morning with others in the building, and they would take a small bus for grocery shopping every week. Mom did OK for about two years, but then she ended up always purchasing the same things over and over again at the store, so we found piles of toilet paper, toothpaste, and other items she'd buy just because she knew them. I found her using deodorant as lotion, and when she put on makeup, it could end up looking pretty comical. We knew she was safe though and slowly added other services like laundry and meals to make sure she was getting everything she needed. It still became hard to get her to wear different clothes, and she started feeling a bit left out at coffee as I think some made fun of her comments. Yes, even seniors can be cruel at times. Mom insisted in telling everyone that she had eaten lunch with Hillary Clinton when she lived in Iowa, but even though she did meet her, the lunch was one of those stories she knew was true but only in her mind.

We moved Mom into the memory care unit on the same summer that I was having chemo. Thus, her mental state had deteriorated quite a bit, though we still tried to have lunch with her every weekend and have her over as much as we could. She still knew us, but her memories were very limited to just a few events that she would repeat over and over again. For some reason, she remembered vividly how the minister had been so scared of falling in the pond when Denny and I got married at the farm. My kids will never forget that story as I think she told it to them multiple times at every meeting. It made me quite sad when I realized how many things she had forgotten when talking with her. I couldn't share all of the wonderful memories of growing up with her as those memories just weren't there for her. I even tried making her famous brownies that she used to bake for all of her women's club meetings, and she swore she had never tasted them before.

Back to the point though, taking care of someone in need is very hard, but there are ways to make things easier. Here are things you should consider:

- Getting medical power of attorney so that you can make medical decisions for others who may not be mentally capable of doing so. Also know if your loved one or friend has a medical directive and what that consists of. Mom would always ask me, "How would I ever know where to go without you?" when going to the doctor or shopping. Sometimes our loved ones or friends just need someone to guide them through life.

- Getting power of attorney to help pay bills and manage accounts.

- Keep good records of everything you do regarding the above so you have them when needed in the future. I keep a fire safe full of file folders with all of Mom's paperwork in it which made things much easier along with tracking all transactions and accounts on a spreadsheet in the computer.

- Consider home assistance such as housekeeping and Meals on Wheels for when you can't be there.

- Label things and write down instructions if your loved one can still read and understand these.

- Don't tell a person with dementia that they are wrong; they just really don't understand.

- Set up automatic delivery of prescriptions if they are still able to know when and how to take these on their own. Mom was actually pretty good at taking the only pill she needed but would sometimes forget to tell me when she ran out. Having this automated helped decrease the last-minute phone calls and runs to the pharmacy.

- Spend time with your loved one, even if it's just to watch TV together or read them a story. My mother always thought she was a poor artist, but she loved the arts-and-crafts pieces that she made in the memory care unit together with others.

- One of the hardest things for us was to convince Mom that she shouldn't be driving anymore. I couldn't believe that she didn't have to take the driver's test when I took her to the DMV. They said that would be age discrimination. Thankfully, in order to park in the underground parking at the senior apartments, the manager made everyone drive with her so she knew they could maneuver through the narrow garage. Mom panicked when her windshield wipers came on and got so flustered that she grudgingly passed over the keys to one of her grandkids. That made our job so much easier, but she didn't let us forget that anytime soon. If you can find someone else to play the "bad guy," that is always helpful.

- Check their pantry and make a surprise care package delivery of things they may need.
- Play music and dance with your loved one. I'll bet you will be rewarded with smiles.
- Know what end-of-life plans your loved one wants and have enough cash on hand to pay for early funeral expenses as needed.

Sometimes you have to make the hard decisions as a caregiver. The hardest decision I've ever had to make was when my mom had a stroke, and I was called upon to say what should happen next. Luckily, I had supportive family members and doctors to talk through everything with, and it was easier knowing that my mother did not want to be kept alive through extensive measures if it meant a life of cognitive impairment and helplessness at the end. I can't say enough good things about the friends, medical staff, and hospice care who supported our family when Mom passed away. In the end, the bumps in my road all have led me to see how important family and friends are in our lives.

I really struggled in sharing the stories of my mother and father, and in no way do I want to dishonor their lives or demean the people they were. My hope is that you will understand that you are not alone, that others have gone through difficult times taking care of those they love, and that you can get through this.

I hope you will consider offering care for a loved one, friend, or even a stranger. The smallest gesture of saying hello or offering a car ride or meal can make a huge impact on someone's life. You'll understand when others are there to help you through the bumps in your road. Welcome the help with open arms.

Appendix A

The Best Advice Others Gave Me

You have to be your own advocate. Be sure to lobby for yourself, ask lots of questions, and have them fit you into their busy schedules. Be prepared to do a lot of paperwork on your own to get lab results, where they need to be and keep a record of everything—you'll want it in the future.

Call the American Cancer Society and ask them for a Personal Health Manager Kit. No one actually told me about this. I inquired about the makeup program that my oncologist told me about, and someone from the American Cancer Society asked if they could send me this organizer. It was a great tool for keeping track of all my paperwork.

My dental hygienist gave me a sample of Biotene for dry mouth. This is great stuff for dry mouth symptoms due to chemo.

Try foods you've never liked before. My sense of taste changed immensely during chemo. Once the first treatment set in, I could really only taste lemon and chocolate. I found that fish, which I really didn't like before, became my favorite food, and I could eat pretty much anything I didn't like the taste of since there simply was no taste.

Ask other breast cancer survivors where they purchased a wig. A friend recommended a great place only fifteen miles from my home. They had over three hundred wigs in stock but only advertised their makeup on the Internet. I never would have found them if I hadn't asked.

Rest when you are tired. After the first chemo session, I went to work but then would come home and take a nap every day. After the second session, I tried pushing myself a little more and soon found that the rest was much needed.

Stay as active as you can be without getting too tired during chemo. Walking, standing, any little movement helps ease the aches and pains a bit.

You may feel pretty good for the first two days after chemo, but then more side effects will set in. For me, I had my first chemotherapy treatments on Friday mornings. Nothing really hit me until that Sunday night, and then my hardest days were Monday and Tuesday. In fact, I went shopping on Saturday, the day after chemo, and had a big family supper after one session too. By Monday morning though, I had to call in sick at work and could only work half a day on Tuesday. By Wednesday, I was able to put a full day's work in but was pretty tired and napped after getting home. Note that I work in an office setting that doesn't require a lot of physical movement or labor.

Prepare a chemo bag with things that you can do to keep your mind off of things during your treatment. I had a just-in-case puke bucket, magazines, pudding, crackers, water, books, and laptop in mine. On the second time, I brought nail polish so my daughter-in-law could paint my nails but probably shouldn't have since the smell was pretty powerful and probably irritated others. Another thing that is irritating is someone who spends the whole time talking on their cell phone while in the infusion room. This is very annoying and rude to others around you.

If you had lymph nodes removed, get a compression sleeve to wear while flying to avoid lymphedema since it can occur at any time, even years after surgery.

Eat and drink water every two hours during chemotherapy to help avoid the nausea. It really works, but sometimes others need to gently remind you of this.

Chemo brain is real. You will easily forget things more during and after chemo, but it gets better.

Neuropathy is also real. This is when your fingers and toes feel numb and tingly. This can be painful at times, but it usually goes away about six weeks after chemotherapy, depending on how many sessions you have to take. I thought that maybe moving my hands and toes a lot would make it go away, but nothing really helps except for certain prescriptions you can get if serious enough.

Appendix B

Things No One Ever Told Me

You can't actually feel the chemicals going into you during a chemotherapy IV drip. I was worried about this and actually asked before my first session since no one had mentioned this during my chemo class. Imagination does strange things to you, and I had all sorts of thoughts of how the chemicals may feel or affect my body as they were going in. No, there is no feeling unless maybe just a chill if the room temperature is cold, but they have warm blankets to keep you comfortable.

They give you great drugs to calm you down during chemo. Though they told us in our chemo class what drugs we'd be getting, they never really told us that the Benadryl would relax you so much that you are in la-la land during the IV drip. That was great.

Surgery and chemotherapy may spark menstruation for women who are not in menopause yet. One of the things that caused me the most aggravation was that on the day of my surgery and each time I had a chemo session, my period would start, and it didn't just make me spot. I had major menstrual periods, each time with heavy bleeding that lasted six to eight days. I was worried about this from the start and proceeded to call my surgeon's nurse when this first happened with my lumpectomy. I asked her, "Is this normal?" She sighed and said that unfortunately, women often respond to trauma by menstruating. How lucky we are! I was still in perimenopause when my journey began, and my oncologist was hoping that chemo would push me into menopause for the follow-up hormone therapy I needed. There were times when I thought it would be much easier to just have a hysterectomy and even asked my oncologist about this as an option.

I only ended up wearing a wig about 20 percent of the time. Otherwise, I found scarves and hats much more comfortable when out in public.

Be very careful in shaving your head with a safety razor. My husband knew how much it was bothering me to have short hair from an electric razor shave catch on chairs and pillows, so he offered to shave my head with his safety razor. I ended up having red bumps all over my head from irritation. If you do this, Burt's Bees baby lotion does help!

Having meals brought in or cooked ahead of time is a godsend, but don't have someone cook meals for you in your own house. My sister Susan is a gem and traveled five hours to be with me during each of my chemo sessions. She was so much help, but I just couldn't tolerate the smell of soups she cooked up to freeze for me. I could take a soup out of the freezer to the microwave to make for a meal, but the smell of anything actually cooking in the house was a real turnoff in eating for me. There was an upside though. If I could force myself to take the first bite, everything was OK after that.

Not everyone in the infusion room where they give the chemotherapy IVs is there for chemo or even for cancer. Some are getting blood, needed nutrients, platelets, etc. You will meet all sorts of people with all sorts of different medical conditions.

The smell of your own excrements for a few days after chemo will be terrible. Yes, this means your urine and bowel movements will have an odor you have never smelled before and you'll never want to smell again. Sometimes this just about made me sick. Helpful hint: Have a room freshener close to the toilet to wave around as needed.

Greeting cards can brighten a survivor's day. It's so hard to know how to help someone who has cancer.

Try just sending a card to cheer them up every so often. It can make a world of difference just knowing there are others who care.

Having assistance with laundry is so nice since you may need to go through more towels and sheets than normal to feel fresh.

There are others out there who suffer from great hot flashes whether from being thrown into menopause from chemotherapy or just naturally. My face gets so hot that it perspires profusely and is often embarrassing. I found some good face antiperspirants online that have really helped slow the perspiring down and have made it much easier to go out in public without having to worry about this embarrassment.

Your doctor will probably recommend getting caught up on all of your vaccinations since chemotherapy and radiation will both run down your immune system. Standard vaccines you will need are for shingles, influenza, and pneumonia.

All those with cancer are eligible to receive a free subscription to "Cure" magazine. I happened across one in the waiting room at the hospital and sent in the postcard for my free copies. I have found this magazine very informative, not only for my own cancer but to keep abreast of new developments in all areas of cancer research. My husband found out he had a slow growing prostate cancer just a year after I was diagnosed with breast cancer so we continue to look for developments in treatments and potential cures.

I never knew a person could be as tired as I was after radiation, and it will last for months afterward as your body is healing. Rest as much as possible.

Regardless if you are a cancer patient or a caregiver, don't feel like you have to be so strong that you don't seek out mental health assistance if you need to. Depression and anxiety are real, and there are things that doctors and other health care professionals can do to help you overcome your feelings. It's OK to have any feeling; it's yours, but you don't have to let it hinder your quality of life.

The most important advice: Don't ever hesitate to ask your friends for help!

Appendix C

I was much honored to be asked to be an honorary chair for our local Relay for Life 2014 "Lights, Cameras, Action." Below is the speech that I gave which I hope will inspire you and others.

Speech for Relay for Life

June 20, 2014

Wow. Thank you so much Kellie Burrows, Kim Poppe, Angie Brown, and the entire team who have rallied for such a great cause and put this year's relay together. Wow. I never expected to be up here speaking as I tend to get pretty nervous in situations like this, and I'll warn you ahead of time that yes, I am a cancer survivor thrown into menopause with those great drugs they have that give you crazy hot flashes, so don't panic and call 911 if I look like I'm starting to melt. I am here tonight to share my story, some tips and tricks that I learned along the way, and I hope a message that you will all hear. I want each and every one of you to know how important you are and that you do make a difference.

I was diagnosed with breast cancer on April 12, 2012, and like my dad who passed away from lung cancer in 1994, I took a very matter-of-fact approach to the whole thing, telling myself that this was just another bump in the road of life. My father wasn't one to lean on anyone else, and I was sure that I could do this all on my own. But as I traveled on in my journey, I found that I needed people in my life now more than ever, and soon, the layers of protection I had built up around myself began to peel away, and this was one of the best things that ever happened to me.

Tonight I'd like to share some of those things that people did for me that helped me get through it. So whether you're a caregiver, a cancer survivor, or just a friend, maybe this will give you some ideas that you can also share with others.

One thing I learned right away was that even though we have a terrific health care system in the United States, you still have to be your own advocate. I was amazed at how I had to call, handcollect, and deliver records between labs, doctors, and hospitals. I really thought that this process would somehow be more seamless and really wondered how someone like my mother, who had suffered dementia, could have managed to get through something like this on her own. I was lucky and did find the greatest nurse at the cancer care unit at the University of Minnesota who made calls for me, set up appointments for me even at other hospitals, made sure she got my records for the doctor, and was there to answer any of my questions—just a phone call away. It was care like this that prompted me to send my surgeon and his team at the U an edible arrangement, and my nurse called to tell me that my surgeon carried the fruit bouquet around the office showing them off to people. Cancer survivors, don't forget that your doctors are people too, and you do make a difference in their lives as much as they make a difference in yours.

Caregivers, please, if you have a chance to go with someone who may need your help at a hospital or clinic, please do so. And ask a lot of questions. Many times, a cancer patient doesn't quite hear everything that the doctor says, so it's really nice to have someone else along to just listen. When I went to chemo class at Regions, I was lucky enough to have my husband with me, but there was a gentleman there, all by himself, and when asked if there would be someone who could drive him to and from his chemo visits, he just replied that he had a sister in California but that she wouldn't be able to come. There are people out there who need you, just to be a friend at times and make that trip with them. Even if you can't make the trip, this is just one thing that you are helping to support just by being here tonight as the American Cancer Society has a great network of volunteers who help drive patients to and from appointments.

I also learned so much about the processes you have to go through from friends at work who had also gone through cancer. It was so nice that they were willing to share their stories with me and let me know what is normal and what to look out for. Cancer survivors, share your stories. Even though they always tell you that everyone is different, these stories help others in their journey and are so important.

The thought of chemotherapy really scared me more than surgery did or even having cancer. I think we all hear about how hard it can be, so I knew I wanted someone with me who wouldn't be too emotional to keep me strong too. When my sister Susan offered to drive up from southern Iowa and go to my first session with me, I jumped on it. My whole family was there for me, but Susan I know could be my rock and would just take care of things. In fact, I would like to dedicate tonight to her as she is here with some of her family, continuing to support me. (Point out Susan.)

Not only did Susan come up for my first chemo session, she came up for each and every one, stayed through those days three and four that seemed to be the worst, cleaned, cooked, did laundry—you name it; she was there to do it. I was a little scared at first when she said she was going to cook for me as we have two other sisters who were really known to be the best cooks in the family. But Susan surprised me, gathered recipes that were supposed to be good for people going through chemo, and actually created some really good meals.

Food is good. Any time you can share prepared meals with a cancer patient, it will always be appreciated. It did bother me sometimes to smell food while it was cooking so bringing a dish in already cooked can be very helpful. Cancer patients going through chemo and radiation may sometimes lose their sense of taste. All I can say is lemon and chocolate. Just about everyone I know who has gone through something similar has said that these are the two things they can actually taste when other foods fall short. I know I ate way more fish with lemon on it during my last rounds of chemo, a habit I probably should have stuck with, but I guess even cancer can't break the Iowa farm girl from her taste for Midwest beef and pork.

Support through chemotherapy can take many forms. Losing your hair is scary, and again, I opted to get help from someone who I knew could get me through this without crying. Jenny, my daughter-in-law, came over with her clippers the day I got out of the shower and had a handful of hair. The trim was good, but my husband convinced me that I wouldn't catch small hairs on my pillow at night if I shaved it all down. Talk about scary—letting my husband take his safety razor to my head. I must have been nuts, but I don't think I ever saw as much love in his eyes as when he was doing this for me.

What else can caregivers do? Care baskets are always nice. A basket of supplies to take to the hospital during an infusion might include magazines, crackers, bottles of water or soda, and an electronic game to play. Though Susan always came up during my treatments,

I had other family members who really wanted to go with me to show their support. It probably wasn't the best idea for Jenny to give me a manicure and pedicure in the infusion room as I think everyone could smell the nail polish, but it did make me feel good and made others smile too. Regions also had their own group of volunteers that would come around with dogs that you could sit and pet and others that would give you a back or foot massage as you were waiting.

My daughter also went with me once, which was a bit scary as she had passed out in elementary school when her class visited the blood bank. The site of most things you may see in a hospital make her queasy, but she held up like a real trooper.

My sister Linda works for a hospice in Venice, Florida, and knew of some great products that were really helpful too. Burt's Bees for Babies lotion and shampoo and Biotene for dry mouth—great stuff.

And don't forget all of the help that the American Cancer Society has to offer. The TLC website offers low-cost hats, wigs, garments, all sorts of things for breast cancer survivors. They also sponsor the Cancer

Legal Line which has sessions all around the Twin Cities to answer questions you may have. Free hats, wigs, and scarves are available through the American Cancer Society, and they also sponsor free makeovers for those going through chemo. Because you are here tonight, your support helps make all of these happen.

One of the best things I got from the American Cancer Society was my Personal Health Manager. This folder is all set up to organize all of your hospital paperwork from appointments, to medications, to bills. Even those simple things make a difference in people's lives.

I never dreamed I could be as tired as I was going through radiation, but I had had a trainer at Life Time Fitness before I got sick and really wanted to get back to working out. Walking back into the gym with very little hair, very little energy, and being totally out of shape was really, really hard; but Krista, Andrea, and all of the trainers there welcomed me back and still comment on how long my hair has gotten. I can even tie it back now.

And I'll come back again to the importance of having a great medical team on your side. No one should ever have to feel uncomfortable going to a doctor. If you do, there's nothing wrong with finding someone else as sometimes people just don't click. I was so lucky to have a great general practitioner to start but then was amazed to find out that I had a whole team of people I could call on—from nurses, to surgeons, to oncologists, to physician assistants, to radiologists, to social workers, to psychologists. Take advantage of the support that is out there. I learned how and can still do self-hypnosis from my psych guy, Scott. That's what I call him. That was a big wall for me to let down— to even think that I needed to talk to a psychologist. I was amazed at how much I've learned about myself in this whole process. Is cancer good? Certainly not, but there are some good things that can come out of the experience, and I encourage you to look for those in your journeys.

I would just like to conclude by letting you know how important you all are and that you do make a difference. You can *light* up someone's life, make those memories that last for the *cameras* in our brains, and please continue to take *action* to help us beat this disease once and for all.

Printed in the United States
By Bookmasters